UNDERSTANDING

RADIO FREQUENCY

SKIN TIGHTENING

FOR BEGINNERS

Enhance Your Beauty Safely:
Effective Rf Treatment Methods, Skin
Rejuvenation Insights, And Expert
Tips For Optimal Results

DR. ALICIA SONYA

CONTENTS

DISCLAIMER

The information provided in this book is for educational and informational purposes only and is not intended as medical advice, diagnosis, or treatment. Always consult with a qualified healthcare professional before beginning any therapy, practice, or lifestyle change.

The author and publisher of this book make no representations or warranties regarding the accuracy, applicability, or completeness of the content presented. While every effort has been made to ensure the information provided is accurate and up-to-date, the field of health and wellness is constantly evolving, and the reader is advised to use discretion and seek professional guidance as needed.

This book contains references to individuals, products, websites, organizations, or other entities solely for informational purposes. The author and publisher do not endorse, sponsor, or affiliate with any of these references, nor do they receive any benefit from their inclusion. The mention of any names, trademarks, or products does not imply any association or endorsement.

The use of this book is solely at the reader's discretion. Neither the author nor the publisher shall be held liable for any damages, loss, or injury resulting from the use or misuse of the information contained herein.

ABOUT THIS BOOK

Understanding Radio Frequency Skin Tightening For Beginners serves as a vital resource for those looking to enhance their understanding of RF skin treatments. With an increase in demand for non-invasive cosmetic procedures, radio-frequency skin tightening has emerged as a popular option for rejuvenating skin without surgery.

This book begins with a comprehensive introduction to RF skin tightening, exploring the science behind how radio frequency energy penetrates skin layers to stimulate collagen production, tighten skin, and reduce signs of aging. Key details on who can benefit most from RF treatments make this guide suitable for anyone curious about enhancing their skin's appearance, while common misconceptions are addressed to ensure readers can approach RF treatments with clarity and confidence.

This book delves deeply into the mechanics of RF technology, explaining how RF energy interacts with skin cells at a foundational level. It covers various types of RF devices, from monopolar to multipolar, each uniquely designed for specific outcomes, such as promoting collagen synthesis or addressing targeted skin layers. Readers gain insights into the safety mechanisms embedded in professional RF devices compared to at-home units, helping to make informed choices on what devices may best serve their needs.

For individuals considering RF treatment, this guide outlines practical aspects of preparation, such as what to expect in a consultation, essential skincare steps before treatment, and how to set realistic expectations. It walks readers through a typical RF session, describing sensations, the duration, and the equipment involved, providing a transparent look at the treatment process.

Additionally, this book outlines differences between professional and at-home RF devices, offering tips for selecting a quality at-home option and maintaining it, while comparing these alternatives to in-office treatments for effectiveness and safety.

Addressing the important topic of safety, this guide informs readers about potential side effects, warning signs that require medical attention, and strategies to minimize irritation or burns. Safety is highlighted particularly for those with sensitive skin, with aftercare recommendations designed to protect and enhance post-treatment outcomes. Post-treatment care is also discussed in depth, emphasizing how specific skincare products, hydration, and sun protection play a crucial role in prolonging RF results, giving readers the tools to extend the benefits of their treatments.

This book also tackles common concerns and questions, such as treatment duration, longevity of results, and cost considerations, along with addressing the suitability of RF for different skin types and areas like the neck and around the eyes. The addition of expert tips from dermatologists and RF technicians provides readers with professional insights, suggesting ways to combine RF treatments with other skincare regimens, adjust routines, and maintain skin elasticity for a lasting youthful glow.

By offering such detailed coverage of RF skin tightening, this guide equips readers with the knowledge and confidence to make informed decisions about their skin health, empowering them to achieve optimal results in their journey toward rejuvenation.

CHAPTER ONE

Introduction To Radio Frequency (RF) Skin Tightening

Radio Frequency (RF) Skin Tightening is a non-invasive cosmetic procedure that uses energy waves to heat the deeper layers of your skin. This heat stimulates collagen and elastin production, two essential proteins that help the skin remain firm and elastic. Over time, collagen in the skin decreases, leading to wrinkles and sagging. RF treatment aims to restore this loss, resulting in a smoother, firmer appearance, often with a single treatment or a short series of sessions.

During the procedure, a specialized device delivers RF energy into the skin's deeper layers, typically penetrating the dermis without affecting the epidermis (outer layer). The heat generated by RF causes minor skin trauma, triggering the body's natural healing process to produce new collagen. This process can be done at a dermatologist's office, aesthetic clinic, or with certain home-use devices, and is usually painless, with some patients experiencing only mild warmth and tingling.

The results of RF skin tightening can vary based on factors like age, skin type, and the device used. Many people start noticing firmer skin within weeks after their first treatment, with continued improvements over several months. It's especially popular for areas prone to sagging, such as the jawline, neck, and around the eyes.

The procedure is widely regarded for its quick recovery time and minimal risk of side effects.

What Is RF Skin Tightening?

RF skin tightening is a technology-driven procedure that targets the skin's inner layers to reduce laxity and improve texture. By delivering radiofrequency waves into the skin, the treatment promotes the production of collagen, which firms and lifts the treated areas. Unlike lasers, which primarily target the skin's surface, RF can penetrate deeper, making it effective for reducing wrinkles and sagging in various skin types and tones.

The treatment itself is usually brief, often lasting between 15-60 minutes depending on the treatment area. A practitioner applies a conductive gel to the skin and then glides the

RF device over the area in slow, circular motions. Patients typically experience mild warmth and a tingling sensation as the device works. There's no downtime, so people can often return to their daily routines immediately after treatment.

RF treatments can be done as a one-time session or as a series for longer-lasting results, depending on individual needs and goals. Results tend to last several months to a few years, particularly when paired with good skincare routine and follow-up sessions every 6-12 months.

It's considered a versatile treatment for those seeking subtle, natural-looking improvements without surgery.

Benefits Of RF Treatment For Skin Rejuvenation

One of the main benefits of RF treatment is its ability to stimulate collagen production, which naturally declines with age. Collagen is key to maintaining skin firmness and elasticity, so by boosting it, RF treatments help improve skin tone and texture. This makes RF particularly beneficial for softening fine lines, lifting the skin around the jawline and neck, and reducing the appearance of wrinkles.

In addition to collagen stimulation, RF treatments offer improved blood circulation in treated areas. Enhanced circulation helps deliver nutrients to the skin, resulting in a radiant and youthful appearance. Some studies suggest that RF can also improve the skin's metabolism, which aids in removing waste products and encourages regeneration, offering a more comprehensive skin-rejuvenating effect.

Another benefit is that RF skin tightening is suitable for all skin types and colors. Unlike some laser treatments, which may pose risks for darker skin tones, RF is safer for a wider range of individuals. The treatment's non-invasive nature and the minimal downtime make it an appealing choice for those who want to avoid surgical lifting procedures but still seek noticeable improvements in skin firmness.

Overview Of How RF Works On Skin

RF works by delivering energy to the skin's deeper layers without affecting the surface.

When RF waves reach the dermis, they produce heat between 40-60°C, depending on the device and desired outcome. This heat stimulates the fibroblast cells that produce collagen and elastin, prompting a rejuvenation process that firms and tightens the skin.

As the skin is heated, it triggers the body's natural repair process, known as controlled thermal injury. This causes a micro-wound response that makes the skin rebuild itself with denser, more organized collagen fibers. Over time, this leads to firmer, more youthful skin.

The results from RF treatments can start becoming visible after a few weeks, as collagen rebuilding continues, and improvements are often fully realized within a few months.

Different RF devices target different depths and intensities, allowing for versatility in treating various skin concerns. For example, monopolar RF can go deeper and is often used for body tightening, while bipolar RF, which is more superficial, is typically used on the face. Understanding these differences helps clients and practitioners tailor the treatment to specific needs.

Suitability: Who Can Benefit From RF Skin Tightening?

RF skin tightening is generally suitable for adults with mild to moderate skin laxity who want to improve their skin tone and firmness without invasive procedures.

It's a popular choice for individuals noticing early signs of aging, such as sagging in the cheeks, jawline, and around the eyes, or those who want to maintain youthful skin. However, those with severe sagging may find more benefit in surgical procedures, as RF offers more subtle and gradual improvements.

People with all skin tones can benefit from RF skin tightening, making it an inclusive treatment. Unlike some other skin treatments, RF doesn't rely on targeting melanin, so it carries a lower risk of hyperpigmentation or burns, even for darker skin tones.

It's also a low-risk option for those unable to undergo laser treatments due to skin sensitivity or who want to avoid the downtime associated with more intensive procedures.

RF is typically not recommended for individuals with pacemakers, metallic implants, or certain skin conditions, as the RF waves can interfere with implants or exacerbate some skin issues. Consulting with a qualified provider is essential to determine if RF is suitable for your skin and health profile. Regular follow-up sessions may be advised for those who want sustained results, usually every 6-12 months.

Myths Vs. Facts About RF Skin Tightening

One common myth is that RF skin tightening results are immediate and last forever. In reality, while some people may see initial results right away, the full effects usually take weeks to months to appear, as collagen production increases gradually.

Additionally, results are not permanent, and follow-up treatments are typically needed to maintain optimal skin firmness over time.

Another misconception is that RF skin tightening can dramatically lift very saggy or loose skin, similar to a surgical facelift. While RF can offer noticeable improvements in firmness and smoothness, it is best suited for mild to moderate laxity. It's a fantastic choice for those seeking subtle enhancement rather than dramatic changes, which are achievable only through surgical interventions.

Lastly, some people fear that RF treatments are painful or unsafe. RF is a low-risk, generally painless procedure, and most patients only feel warmth or mild tingling.

The technology has been FDA-approved and tested for safety and efficacy. As long as the treatment is performed by a qualified provider, RF skin tightening is a reliable and safe option for rejuvenating and tightening skin.

CHAPTER TWO

Understanding How RF Technology Works

Radiofrequency (RF) technology for skin tightening uses low-energy waves to heat the deeper layers of the skin, targeting the dermis without damaging the outer layer, or epidermis. The RF waves cause a controlled injury to collagen fibers, making them contract. This process not only provides an immediate tightening effect but also initiates collagen production, which improves skin elasticity and firmness over time. The technique is suitable for various areas of the body, including the face, neck, and arms.

To perform RF skin tightening, a practitioner typically applies a conductive gel to the skin, which helps transmit the RF waves smoothly. An RF device, either handheld or mounted, is then moved across the targeted skin areas. This heating process may be felt as warmth, but most devices have adjustable settings to ensure comfort, with sessions typically lasting between 15 to 45 minutes depending on the area.

Many people opt for RF skin tightening because it's a non-invasive method with minimal recovery time. Unlike more invasive cosmetic procedures, RF technology works gradually, with most users experiencing improved skin tone and reduced fine lines over several weeks as collagen builds. Optimal results usually require multiple sessions, spaced a few weeks apart.

Basic Science: How RF Energy Affects Skin

RF energy affects the skin by gently heating the dermis, the middle layer of skin, which triggers a response from fibroblasts—cells responsible for collagen and elastin production. When fibroblasts detect this heat, they signal the body to create more collagen fibers to "repair" the slight thermal injury. This increase in collagen supports the skin's structure, reduces fine lines, and improves skin elasticity.

The thermal effect from RF energy also breaks down existing, weak collagen fibers, which are then replaced by stronger, new collagen. This heat-induced collagen remodeling process can take several weeks, and the changes are usually gradual.

As more sessions are completed, the skin becomes firmer, and wrinkles and fine lines soften, making the skin look more youthful and smooth.

RF energy is particularly effective because it is precise, delivering heat only to specific depths within the skin without damaging the epidermis. This selective energy application is safe and efficient, making RF skin tightening a reliable choice for many who seek non-invasive rejuvenation.

Different Types Of RF Devices And Their Purposes

RF skin tightening can be performed using various types of devices, each serving specific needs. Monopolar RF devices are often used in professional settings as they penetrate deeply, providing effective results on larger areas like the abdomen or thighs. These devices use a single electrode to deliver RF energy into the skin, reaching the deeper layers effectively.

Bipolar RF devices, on the other hand, have two electrodes and are commonly used for facial skin tightening as they provide more controlled heating. Because they target shallower layers, bipolar devices are ideal for treating fine lines and mild sagging. Additionally, multipolar RF devices combine multiple electrodes to allow even distribution of heat, which can provide faster and more comfortable sessions for larger skin areas.

For at-home use, many manufacturers offer handheld RF devices that provide less intense

RF energy to ensure safety. These are suitable for maintaining professional results between sessions and can be used on smaller areas like the face and neck. However, they're generally less powerful than devices used in clinical settings, making them more suitable for mild to moderate tightening effects.

Collagen Production And RF: How It's Stimulated

RF energy stimulates collagen production by heating the dermal layer, which activates fibroblasts to begin collagen synthesis. The RF waves generate mild thermal stress, tricking the skin into a "repair mode," where it naturally produces collagen and elastin, essential proteins for skin structure and elasticity. This process tightens and firms skin, improving texture and reducing fine lines.

Collagen production continues for weeks after an RF treatment, as fibroblasts remain active. By scheduling regular RF sessions, collagen levels are sustained, allowing for cumulative tightening and rejuvenating effects over time. For best results, most practitioners recommend a series of treatments spaced one month apart to allow new collagen to stabilize and build up.

The results of RF treatments are subtle but gradually noticeable. Collagen acts as the skin's framework, so as it replenishes, the skin gains firmness and resilience.

Users experience smoother skin texture and improved tone as collagen density increases, making RF an effective and non-invasive choice for long-term skin health.

Safety Mechanisms In RF Devices

RF devices come with built-in safety mechanisms to protect the skin from overheating or injury. Most RF devices include temperature sensors that monitor the skin's surface, adjusting the energy output if the device detects excessive heat. This feature ensures that the treatment remains comfortable and that the skin is not overheated, which could cause burns.

Many professional RF devices also have automatic cutoffs or cooling elements. These cooling features protect the outer skin while allowing the dermis to reach the necessary temperature for collagen stimulation. Some devices even include preset modes for different skin types or areas of the body, optimizing safety and effectiveness for each individual.

At-home RF devices are generally designed with lower energy levels and additional safety features, like reduced heat levels and automatic timers, to prevent overuse. The intention behind these features is to ensure that even inexperienced users can safely use RF treatments in the comfort of their homes, with minimal risk of adverse effects.

Key Components In Professional Vs. At-Home RF Devices

Professional RF devices are often larger, more powerful, and built to handle various skin types and treatment areas. They typically include adjustable settings, temperature control, and multiple attachments to cater to different body areas, such as the face, neck, or abdomen. These devices are used by trained practitioners who understand the optimal energy levels needed for effective collagen stimulation.

At-home RF devices are generally smaller, easier to operate, and less intense. They are usually handheld, with simpler controls to make them safe for casual users. Though they deliver less energy than professional devices, they are effective for minor skin-tightening results and maintaining professional outcomes between clinic sessions. These devices are typically cordless, allowing users the flexibility to treat their skin wherever convenient.

In both professional and at-home RF devices, essential components include an RF emitter and a cooling mechanism, which work together to deliver energy safely. Professional devices may also incorporate LED light therapy or ultrasound to enhance results, while at-home devices focus on user-friendly designs to encourage regular use without the need for specialized training.

CHAPTER THREE

Types Of RF Treatments

Radio Frequency (RF) skin tightening treatments vary widely, and each type uses specific techniques to rejuvenate and firm the skin. Traditional RF treatments focus on heating the skin to stimulate collagen and elastin production, essential for skin elasticity. These treatments use different levels of heat penetration, depending on the device and approach, to treat various skin concerns effectively. Some treatments are best suited for surface-level issues, while others target deeper layers of the skin.

Professional RF treatments include in-office procedures, where dermatologists or estheticians use advanced RF machines to achieve effective and longer-lasting results. At-home RF devices are also available for more convenient options, although they're typically less potent. Patients often choose in-office treatments for faster, more visible outcomes, while at-home devices are suitable for maintenance.

RF skin tightening also varies based on how it interacts with the skin. While some RF treatments only heat the top layers, others go deeper to treat wrinkles and tighten skin tissue comprehensively.

The duration of results depends on the frequency and type of RF treatment, with most options requiring multiple sessions for optimal results.

Monopolar, Bipolar, And Multipolar RF Explained

Monopolar RF uses a single electrode to deliver energy deep into the skin, reaching the dermis and subcutaneous layers. It is highly effective for treating sagging skin and larger areas, like the neck or stomach, where deeper penetration is necessary. Monopolar RF is common in professional settings because of its intensity and ability to stimulate significant collagen production, offering more dramatic skin-tightening results.

Bipolar RF, in contrast, uses two electrodes to create energy in the top layer of the skin. The shallower penetration is ideal for fine lines, slight wrinkles, and surface rejuvenation. It is less intense than monopolar, making it more suitable for sensitive skin areas, such as around the eyes. Bipolar RF is also often found in home devices, as it's safe and simple to use without professional supervision.

Multipolar RF incorporates three or more electrodes to deliver RF energy with greater precision and control, making it versatile for both deep and surface-level treatments. It heats the skin evenly and comfortably, often used for facial treatments to enhance skin texture, elasticity, and firmness.

Many prefer multipolar RF for its balanced effects on both superficial and deeper skin layers, offering comprehensive tightening with reduced discomfort.

Fractional RF: What It Is And Its Benefits
Fractional RF technology breaks the energy into smaller, targeted segments, focusing on

specific skin areas without affecting the surrounding tissue. This method allows for controlled, precise treatment of problem areas, like acne scars, deep wrinkles, and uneven skin texture. Fractional RF's pinpoint accuracy makes it ideal for reducing downtime, as it minimizes skin irritation and supports faster recovery.

In addition to improving skin texture, fractional RF stimulates significant collagen production, which helps in firming the skin and improving elasticity. It works by delivering heat only to tiny portions of the skin, which boosts healing and skin cell turnover, resulting in smoother and tighter skin. This is a preferred option for individuals seeking less invasive options with noticeable results over time.

Fractional RF treatments generally require multiple sessions for optimal results, spaced a few weeks apart. Each session builds on the previous one, allowing gradual yet long-lasting improvements. Because it treats specific areas, fractional RF is highly adaptable for all skin types and is effective for both anti-aging and skin-rejuvenation purposes, delivering targeted results without extensive damage.

Micro-Needling With RF: An Advanced Approach

Micro-needling with RF combines the collagen-boosting effects of micro-needling with the skin-tightening power of RF energy.

During this treatment, tiny needles penetrate the skin's surface, creating micro-injuries that stimulate natural healing and collagen production. As the needles reach deeper layers, RF energy is simultaneously delivered to intensify collagen production and improve skin elasticity.

The dual-action technique is highly effective for treating wrinkles, fine lines, acne scars, and even stretch marks. Unlike traditional micro-needling, which affects only the surface, RF micro-needling heats the skin below the surface, resulting in firmer, smoother skin with more significant tightening effects. This treatment is particularly beneficial for areas with severe signs of aging, as the combination boosts collagen production more effectively than either treatment alone.

Sessions typically last about 30 to 45 minutes, and results are gradual, improving over several months as the skin continues to heal and regenerate. Most people require three to four sessions, spaced one month apart, to achieve desired results. Micro-needling with RF is known for its long-lasting effects and suitability for multiple skin issues, offering a powerful option for skin rejuvenation.

Comparing RF With Ultrasound And Laser Treatments

RF skin tightening is often compared with ultrasound and laser treatments, as each technique offers unique advantages for skin rejuvenation.

RF uses radiofrequency energy to heat the skin, while ultrasound treatments use sound waves, and lasers rely on light energy. RF is known for its ability to treat deeper layers without damaging the surface, making it versatile for skin tightening without significant downtime.

Ultrasound treatments, like HIFU (High-Intensity Focused Ultrasound), penetrate even deeper than RF and are particularly effective for lifting the skin, especially in areas like the neck and jawline.

HIFU is ideal for patients seeking subtle, natural-looking lift effects and is often used as a non-surgical facelift. However, it may be less effective on surface-level skin concerns like fine lines and pigmentation.

Laser treatments focus primarily on the skin's surface, making them excellent for treating sun damage, pigmentation, and fine wrinkles. Unlike RF and ultrasound, lasers require more caution on darker skin tones due to potential pigmentation risks.

Each method has unique strengths, and choosing between them depends on skin type, target issues, and desired outcome, with RF being the most versatile for comprehensive tightening.

Choosing The Right Type For Your Skin Goals

Selecting the ideal RF treatment depends on individual skin concerns, goals, and skin type. For targeting deep wrinkles, sagging skin, or larger areas like the abdomen, monopolar or multipolar RF treatments are typically the best choice due to their intense, far-reaching effects. Those with mild skin laxity or fine lines may find bipolar RF more suitable for superficial tightening and rejuvenation.

For people with specific problem areas, fractional RF is highly effective, especially for acne scars, uneven skin texture, and deeper wrinkles. It focuses energy on targeted points, minimizing downtime and skin irritation. RF micro-needling, on the other hand, is recommended for those needing extensive rejuvenation for both surface and deeper skin layers, addressing issues like stretch marks, scars, and loose skin with precision.

Ultimately, consulting with a licensed provider ensures a tailored approach to RF treatment, as they can recommend options based on unique skin goals. Factors like downtime, intensity, and desired results play a role in choosing the most effective RF type, helping to achieve optimal skin tightening and rejuvenation with minimal risks and tailored results.

CHAPTER FOUR

Preparing For Your First RF Treatment

To ensure the best experience with your radio frequency (RF) skin tightening treatment, preparing adequately is essential. Start by cleaning your face thoroughly before your appointment, and removing all makeup, lotions, and sunscreen. This ensures the RF device can work directly on your skin without interference.

Hydrate well in the days leading up to your appointment—drinking water helps boost your skin's elasticity, which can improve treatment results. Many professionals also recommend avoiding direct sun exposure a few days before the treatment, as sunburned or irritated skin can become more sensitive to RF energy and may react poorly.

It's also important to understand that this process works gradually, so a series of sessions is typically required for optimal results. On average, clients may need about 6 to 12 sessions, spaced 1-2 weeks apart, to notice significant changes. RF skin tightening doesn't produce drastic immediate results; rather, it encourages collagen production over time. This helps create a naturally firmer, smoother skin appearance as new collagen builds up over the weeks following treatment.

For your first session, plan to arrive at the clinic about 15 minutes early, allowing you time to relax and fill out any necessary forms. Wear loose, comfortable clothing to avoid any irritation post-treatment, especially if RF will be applied to areas like the neck or body. Remember that RF skin tightening has minimal downtime, so you should be able to return to regular activities soon after, though avoiding intense heat (such as saunas) for 24-48 hours is recommended.

Consultation And Skin Analysis: What To Expect

During your consultation, the specialist will assess your skin type, tone, and elasticity to determine the suitability of RF treatment for your needs. This is a chance to discuss your skincare concerns, medical history, and any previous treatments you've undergone. The skin analysis may involve a close visual inspection or the use of a digital imaging device to provide a comprehensive view of your skin's underlying layers, which can help the provider customize the treatment.

The specialist will explain how RF skin tightening works, discussing how radio frequency energy heats the skin layers to encourage collagen production and achieve a tightening effect. Based on your skin analysis, they'll recommend a treatment plan tailored to your skin's specific needs, including the number of sessions and the frequency of treatments required. For areas needing significant tightening, such as around the eyes or jowls, a more frequent treatment schedule might be suggested initially, followed by maintenance sessions.

Ask questions about the treatment to clarify any uncertainties you might have. This is the ideal time to understand realistic outcomes and address any concerns. Your provider should be transparent about potential side effects, such as mild redness or swelling, so you can make an informed decision. This consultation phase helps you build trust with your provider and ensures that you feel comfortable and well-prepared for the upcoming sessions.

Essential Pre-Treatment Skincare Steps

A few days before your RF skin tightening session, begin following a gentle skincare routine to prepare your skin. This includes using a mild cleanser that maintains the skin's pH balance, along with a lightweight moisturizer to keep your skin hydrated. Avoid any abrasive exfoliants or scrubs, as they can leave your skin more sensitive to the RF device. It's also beneficial to avoid any active ingredients in your skincare, such as retinoids or vitamin C, in the 2-3 days leading up to the treatment.

Sun protection is critical during this period. Apply a broad-spectrum sunscreen with an SPF of 30 or higher, especially if you'll be outside, as RF treatment on sun-damaged skin can increase sensitivity. Hydrating sheet masks or soothing serums can also help create an optimal environment for your skin by ensuring it's well-moisturized but not greasy. Some clinics may also recommend hydrating serums containing hyaluronic acid, which binds moisture to the skin and enhances the treatment outcome.

Finally, consider limiting caffeine and alcohol intake, as these can dehydrate the skin and reduce its elasticity. Opt for plenty of water, herbal teas, or hydrating foods like cucumbers and watermelon. Avoiding caffeine and alcohol also helps reduce any potential inflammation or sensitivity during treatment, allowing your skin to respond more favorably to the RF energy.

Products To Avoid Before RF Treatment

Several skincare products should be avoided to prevent any adverse skin reactions during RF treatment. First, discontinue the use of any exfoliating acids, such as glycolic or salicylic acid, at least 3 days before your appointment, as these can make your skin more sensitive.

Retinoids, including retinol and tretinoin, should also be paused around 3-5 days in advance. These ingredients can cause dryness or peeling, increasing the risk of irritation when RF energy is applied.

Avoid using any topical treatments containing benzoyl peroxide, a common ingredient in acne treatments, as it can dry out the skin and heighten sensitivity to RF. Vitamin C serums, although great for brightening skin, are another product to skip in the days leading up to RF, as they can make the skin more reactive to heat. Stick to simple, gentle moisturizing products that don't contain active ingredients.

Be cautious about essential oils or fragrances in your skincare as well, as they may trigger skin reactions when combined with RF.

Your goal is to maintain a calm, well-hydrated base that will respond optimally to treatment. Consulting with your skincare provider can help identify any specific products you might need to avoid based on your unique skin type and needs.

What To Wear And Bring To Your Appointment

Choosing the right attire for your RF skin tightening appointment can make the process more comfortable. Opt for loose, breathable clothing, particularly if you'll be receiving treatment on areas beyond the face, such as the neck or body.

Avoid tight necklines or fitted tops, as these could irritate treated skin. If you're having facial RF, consider wearing a button-down shirt or a top that's easy to remove without touching the face.

To protect your skin after treatment, bring along a wide-brimmed hat and sunglasses if you're having a facial treatment, as sun exposure immediately after RF can lead to increased sensitivity. It's also a good idea to bring a water bottle to stay hydrated throughout the day—hydration plays a key role in supporting collagen synthesis after treatment.

Since RF skin tightening may leave your skin slightly flushed, having a mild moisturizer or soothing gel on hand can also be beneficial for calming the skin post-treatment.

Some clinics may offer topical cooling or soothing treatments after RF, but you can always bring your gentle skincare product if you prefer.

For instance, a calming aloe gel can help ease any warmth or mild irritation after the session. Avoid makeup immediately after treatment, so plan to go makeup-free to your appointment or bring a makeup bag if you'll need to reapply before leaving.

Understanding And Setting Realistic Expectations

Setting realistic expectations is crucial for satisfaction with RF skin-tightening results. This treatment provides gradual results as it stimulates natural collagen production, so don't expect dramatic changes after a single session. Generally, visible improvements begin to appear after 4-6 sessions, with the skin feeling firmer and smoother over time. The treatment is designed to lift and tighten, but it's important to remember that results vary based on age, skin type, and lifestyle factors.

The improvements you experience with RF skin tightening can last anywhere from six months to two years with proper aftercare and maintenance. Many people choose to have follow-up sessions every 6-12 months to maintain the results, as collagen production naturally slows with age. Combining RF skin tightening with other complementary treatments, like microneedling or chemical peels, may also help enhance results over time, depending on your skincare goals.

It's also important to understand that RF skin tightening won't deliver the same results as surgical procedures. However, it provides a non-invasive alternative that's low-risk, with minimal discomfort and downtime. The treatment is suitable for those looking to rejuvenate their skin subtly and naturally without extensive recovery periods.

CHAPTER FIVE

Step-By-Step RF Treatment Procedure

Radiofrequency (RF) skin tightening starts with skin preparation to ensure it is clean and free from any oils or dirt that could interfere with the process. The practitioner typically cleanses the area to be treated and may apply a conductive gel to help the RF device glide smoothly. Once the skin is prepared, the RF device is set to the appropriate temperature and intensity, tailored to the skin type and treatment area.

Next, the practitioner begins moving the RF device over the target areas in circular or sweeping motions, ensuring even coverage and maintaining contact with the skin.

This part of the procedure takes anywhere from 10 to 30 minutes per area, depending on the size of the treatment zone. The goal is to achieve a gradual warming of the dermal layers without overheating, which stimulates collagen production for skin tightening.

After the entire area has been treated, the practitioner removes any remaining gel, and a soothing cream or moisturizer is often applied to minimize any redness or irritation. This final step helps to lock in moisture and promotes skin healing.

There's generally no need for downtime after RF treatment, though practitioners may recommend avoiding direct sunlight or strenuous exercise for 24 hours.

What Happens During An RF Session

During an RF skin tightening session, the practitioner begins by positioning the patient comfortably and explaining the steps involved in the treatment. Once the skin is prepped, they adjust the RF device settings based on the patient's skin type and the desired results. Typically, the practitioner will start with a low temperature and gradually increase it to an optimal level where the skin reaches a mild warmth, which encourages collagen production.

The device is then passed over the target areas in a systematic pattern, ensuring that the heat penetrates evenly. Patients usually feel a warm sensation as the device moves, with some experiencing mild tingling.

The practitioner monitors the skin's response and adjusts the settings as needed to prevent any discomfort or potential skin damage. The treatment duration varies based on the area and skin needs, but each session generally lasts between 30 to 60 minutes.

As the session concludes, the practitioner may assess the skin for any signs of irritation and apply a post-treatment serum or moisturizer. This step helps soothe the skin and reduce any mild redness.

Patients are encouraged to keep the treated area moisturized and avoid strong sun exposure for a day or two to ensure optimal healing and collagen formation.

Key Tools And Equipment Used In RF Procedures

The primary tool in RF skin tightening is the RF device, which comes in various forms depending on the treatment area and method. Handheld devices for at-home treatments are available, but professional-grade machines in clinics often deliver more consistent results. These machines typically feature adjustable temperature and power settings to tailor the treatment to individual skin types, minimizing risks of burns or irritation.

Most RF devices require a conductive gel to ensure smooth movement and proper heat penetration into the dermal layers. The gel not only reduces friction but also helps control temperature distribution across the treatment area. Other equipment, such as cooling mechanisms or contact thermometers, may be used to keep the skin at a safe temperature throughout the session.

Finally, post-treatment products like soothing creams or anti-inflammatory serums are often applied after the procedure. These products aid in calming the skin, promoting hydration, and maximizing the treatment's effectiveness. With a combination of quality RF devices and professional-grade aftercare products, practitioners ensure both immediate comfort and long-term skin-tightening benefits.

Pain And Sensation: What You'll Experience

RF treatments are generally non-invasive and well-tolerated by most patients, with sensations mainly involving mild heat or warmth on the skin. The heat can feel similar to a warm massage, which is comfortable for many people, although sensitive areas may produce a slight tingling or prickling sensation. The practitioner controls these sensations by adjusting the device's intensity, so most patients experience minimal discomfort.

In rare cases, patients with lower pain thresholds may feel mild discomfort as the heat builds up during longer treatments. For this reason, it's crucial to communicate openly with the practitioner if any pain or excessive heat is felt, so adjustments can be made. The conductive gel applied before treatment also helps to minimize any potential discomfort by distributing heat evenly and cooling the skin's surface.

After the session, patients may notice minor redness or warmth in the treated area, which usually subsides within a few hours. Unlike some other cosmetic treatments, RF skin tightening does not typically cause swelling or bruising. Using a gentle moisturizer can help soothe any post-treatment sensations and promote quicker recovery, leaving patients comfortable and refreshed after their session.

Duration Of Treatment And Aftercare Advice

RF skin tightening sessions usually last between 30 to 60 minutes per area, depending on the size and needs of the treatment zone.

Larger areas like the abdomen or thighs may require longer sessions, while smaller facial areas can often be completed in 15 to 30 minutes. Practitioners often recommend a series of treatments, typically spaced about 2 to 4 weeks apart, to maximize collagen production and long-term results.

After the session, it's advisable to follow basic aftercare steps to help the skin heal and optimize the procedure's effects. Avoiding direct sun exposure for the first 24 hours is essential, as the skin can be more sensitive to UV rays immediately after treatment. Applying a gentle moisturizer helps soothe the skin and maintain hydration, promoting faster recovery and enhancing the skin's elasticity.

Practitioners may also advise patients to avoid heavy workouts or saunas for a day, as excessive heat could interfere with the treatment's benefits. With each successive session, the skin's texture and firmness typically improve, creating cumulative results that can last up to a year. Proper aftercare, including consistent hydration and sun protection, will prolong the tightening effects of RF treatments.

Immediate Results Vs. Long-Term Effects

RF skin tightening treatments offer both immediate and long-term benefits. Many patients notice an initial tightening and smoothing effect immediately after the session, as the heat causes collagen fibers to contract.

This temporary effect gives the skin a slightly firmer, lifted appearance that is most visible within the first few hours post-treatment, especially around areas with finer lines.

The long-term benefits develop as the body gradually produces new collagen in response to the controlled heat exposure. Over the weeks following treatment, patients often notice improvements in skin elasticity, texture, and overall firmness. This natural collagen production process helps the skin retain a more youthful appearance and diminishes the look of wrinkles or sagging over time.

For optimal, sustained results, practitioners typically recommend multiple sessions, as repeated treatments build up collagen levels and enhance skin firmness.

With proper maintenance and occasional follow-up treatments, these effects can last for six months to a year, providing patients with a more enduring solution to skin laxity than many other non-invasive methods.

CHAPTER SIX

At-Home RF Skin Tightening Devices

Radio Frequency (RF) skin tightening devices are non-invasive tools that use energy waves to heat the deeper layers of the skin. This process encourages collagen and elastin production, reducing fine lines and sagging skin. At-home RF devices are smaller, portable versions of professional machines, designed to allow users to perform treatments conveniently without needing a clinic visit. These devices typically target the face, neck, arms, and other areas prone to aging.

To use an at-home RF device, apply a conductive gel to the target area to ensure even heat distribution and prevent discomfort.

Gently glide the device in circular motions on the skin, focusing on problem areas. Most devices come with preset energy levels—begin at a low setting and gradually increase as you grow comfortable. Treatments usually last 10–20 minutes per area, depending on the device.

Consistency is key to achieving results with RF devices. Regular treatments, often 2-3 times a week for the first few months, help rebuild collagen over time.

Improvements may become visible after 6–8 weeks, with the skin looking firmer and more lifted. Always follow the manufacturer's guidelines to avoid overuse or skin irritation.

Choosing A Quality At-Home RF Device

When choosing a quality RF skin-tightening device, it's essential to focus on safety features, energy levels, and device certifications. Look for devices with FDA approval or CE marking, ensuring they meet safety standards. Models offering multiple heat settings allow better customization to match your skin type and treatment goals.

Research customer reviews and seek devices from reputable brands with proven results. Devices with ergonomic designs and intuitive controls make at-home treatments easier and more comfortable.

Consider whether the machine comes with accessories, such as gels or storage cases, that enhance the user experience.

Battery life and portability are also important if you plan to travel with the device. Devices with rechargeable batteries are more convenient than corded ones, especially for frequent users. Be sure to purchase from authorized retailers to avoid counterfeit products, which may pose safety risks.

Tips For Safe And Effective At-Home Treatments

To ensure safe and effective RF treatments, always start by cleaning your skin thoroughly to remove makeup, dirt, or oils.

Apply a thin layer of conductive gel before treatment to prevent skin burns and ensure smooth gliding of the device. Avoid treating areas with open wounds, active acne, or sensitive skin conditions.

Begin with shorter sessions and lower heat settings to assess how your skin responds. Gradually increase the energy level as you grow accustomed to the device. Follow the recommended frequency in the instruction manual—most devices suggest 2–3 treatments per week initially.

After each session, moisturize your skin to lock in hydration and enhance results. Avoid sun exposure or apply sunscreen if you've treated areas prone to UV sensitivity. If any redness or discomfort occurs, reduce the intensity or frequency of use to avoid irritation.

Comparing At-Home RF To Professional Treatments

While at-home RF devices offer convenience and affordability, professional RF treatments deliver more powerful and quicker results. In-office procedures are performed using medical-grade equipment operated by trained professionals, making them more effective for severe skin laxity and deep wrinkles.

At-home devices, though less potent, are ideal for maintenance and early signs of aging. They provide gradual improvements, which are well-suited for users with mild skin concerns. Treatments at home are also time-saving since they avoid clinic visits and allow for flexible scheduling.

However, professional treatments come with higher costs and may require multiple sessions. If you need significant results for special events, a professional procedure might be preferable. But for ongoing care and prevention, at-home RF devices are an excellent option.

Maintenance And Care Of Your Device

Proper maintenance of your RF device ensures it remains effective and safe to use. After every session, clean the device head with a soft cloth or disinfecting wipe to remove residual gel and dirt. Avoid using water unless the manual states it's safe, as moisture can damage the internal components.

Store the device in a cool, dry place away from direct sunlight. If it comes with a storage case, use it to prevent dust buildup and accidental damage. Recharge the battery regularly to avoid interruptions during your sessions, especially if the device is used frequently.

Routine inspections help ensure the device stays in good condition. Look out for frayed cords, damaged parts, or malfunctioning buttons. Contact the manufacturer's customer service for repairs if needed. Keeping the device well-maintained can extend its lifespan and improve long-term results.

Budget-Friendly Options Vs. Premium Devices

Budget-friendly RF devices offer basic functionality at a lower cost, making them an attractive option for beginners. These models typically provide fewer energy levels and features but can still deliver gradual results with consistent use. They are ideal for those looking to test RF treatments before investing in higher-end devices.

Premium devices, on the other hand, come with advanced features like multiple heat settings, LED therapy modes, or app integration for progress tracking. They often provide better ergonomics, faster results, and improved safety features, making them suitable for more serious users.

When deciding between budget and premium devices, consider your skin care goals, frequency of use, and budget. While high-end devices may offer faster outcomes, budget options can still be effective with patience and regular treatments.

Reading reviews and comparing specifications helps you find the best fit for your needs.

CHAPTER SEVEN

RF Skin Tightening Safety And Side Effects

Radiofrequency (RF) skin tightening uses RF energy to heat the skin's deeper layers, stimulating collagen production for firmer skin. While the procedure is generally safe, users should understand potential risks and side effects.

Common side effects include mild redness, swelling, or tingling immediately after treatment, which usually subsides within hours to a few days. This response is typical and indicates the skin is responding to the controlled RF energy. Maintaining clear communication with your provider can ensure your skin is monitored, especially if it is your first session.

For a safe treatment experience, it's important to be honest with your provider about any skin sensitivities, medical conditions, or recent skin treatments, as these can influence how your skin reacts to RF energy. During the procedure, technicians use protective gel and carefully monitor the skin's temperature to avoid excessive heating. This control is crucial in preventing more serious effects like burns or hyperpigmentation, particularly for those with darker skin tones.

Preparation is essential for a smooth process. Avoid skin-irritating products, direct sun exposure, or any form of exfoliation in the days leading up to treatment.

Post-treatment, avoid touching or irritating the skin, wear sunscreen, and moisturize to aid recovery. Regular follow-ups can help assess skin response and adjust treatment if necessary.

Common Side Effects And How To Manage Them

Common side effects of RF skin tightening include redness, swelling, and minor discomfort, typically mild and temporary. Redness may be visible immediately after treatment, but it should fade within a few hours to a day.

Swelling is another potential reaction, though it generally lessens by using cold compresses or soothing gels applied directly to the treated area.

These side effects are a normal part of the body's natural response to collagen-stimulating treatments.

To manage these effects, cool compresses and soothing moisturizers (like aloe vera) are effective. Avoid harsh cleansers or exfoliating products for a few days post-treatment, as these can irritate the skin further. Keeping the skin hydrated is essential, so drink plenty of water and use gentle, fragrance-free moisturizers to help soothe and repair the skin.

In some cases, clients may notice slight peeling or dryness as the skin regenerates. This can be managed with gentle moisturizers and avoiding products with active ingredients like retinol or AHAs until the skin fully recovers. Maintaining a consistent post-treatment routine helps manage side effects while supporting the skin's healing process.

Warning Signs: When To Seek Medical Attention

Though RF skin tightening is safe, certain symptoms should be closely monitored. Severe pain, blisters, intense swelling, or prolonged redness are not typical and may indicate a reaction requiring medical attention. Blistering could result from improper device settings or individual sensitivity, and it's essential to notify your provider or seek medical advice if this occurs to prevent scarring or infection.

If you notice persistent itching, a rash, or changes in skin texture that worsen rather than improve, this could be a sign of an adverse reaction. Some individuals may experience allergic responses to the topical products used before or after treatment, so discussing any sensitivities with your provider beforehand can help minimize these risks.

Another warning sign is hyperpigmentation, especially in individuals with darker skin tones, as they are more prone to this issue. If you experience darkening or lightening of the skin that lasts beyond a few weeks, consult a dermatologist to discuss treatments for pigmentation.

Proactive monitoring of these warning signs can ensure timely intervention and minimize long-term effects.

Avoiding Burns And Irritation During RF Treatments

Burns during RF treatments are rare but can occur if devices are used incorrectly or if settings are too high. Before beginning, it's essential to ensure the practitioner is certified and experienced in RF skin treatments. They should assess your skin type and adjust device settings accordingly to avoid overheating. Using a conductive gel also helps to distribute the RF energy evenly, reducing the risk of burns and enhancing comfort.

Temperature monitoring throughout the treatment is vital. Many devices have built-in temperature controls, but experienced practitioners also frequently assess your skin's temperature to ensure comfort and safety.

If you feel excessive heat or discomfort during treatment, communicate this immediately so adjustments can be made.

Proper skin preparation is another preventive measure. Avoid exfoliating treatments, harsh skincare products, or direct sun exposure beforehand, as these can make skin more sensitive to heat. A well-prepared, well-monitored treatment ensures that you get the benefits of RF skin tightening without unwanted burns or irritation.

Safety Tips For Sensitive Skin Types

If you have sensitive skin, RF skin tightening can still be safe if done with extra caution. Inform your provider about your skin's sensitivity, as they can adjust the settings accordingly.

Using a lower frequency or shorter treatment duration helps reduce irritation for sensitive skin. This approach ensures that the skin benefits from the collagen-stimulating effects without experiencing excessive discomfort.

Patch testing is a good precautionary step for sensitive skin types. Before a full treatment, ask for a small trial area to gauge your skin's reaction. If there's no adverse response, you can proceed with a full session confidently. Additionally, consider scheduling sessions with longer intervals between them to give your skin adequate recovery time.

After treatment, sensitive skin requires special care. Use gentle cleansers, avoid hot water, and apply a soothing, fragrance-free moisturizer to aid recovery.

Reducing sun exposure and applying a broad-spectrum sunscreen daily is also crucial for maintaining results and protecting sensitive skin from potential post-treatment discoloration.

Proper Aftercare To Minimize Risks

Post-treatment aftercare is crucial to ensuring safe and lasting results with RF skin tightening. For the first 24-48 hours after treatment, avoid touching or rubbing the treated area to prevent irritation or infection. Keeping the skin clean with a gentle, fragrance-free cleanser and following with a hydrating moisturizer can aid the skin's recovery and help lock in moisture.

Sun protection is particularly important following RF skin tightening.

The treatment makes the skin more vulnerable to UV damage, so wearing broad-spectrum SPF 30 or higher daily will protect against hyperpigmentation and premature aging. Avoid excessive heat, such as saunas or hot showers, for a few days, as this can increase redness and slow healing.

Following a routine of hydration, gentle care, and sun protection maximizes the benefits of RF skin tightening while minimizing any potential side effects.

Consistency in aftercare not only enhances results but also protects your skin's health, ensuring smoother and firmer skin without the risk of complications.

CHAPTER EIGHT

Optimizing Results With Post-Treatment Care

After a radio frequency (RF) skin tightening session, taking care of your skin can significantly enhance and extend the results. Post-treatment, your skin may feel warm and slightly sensitive; therefore, it's essential to avoid touching or irritating the treated areas. Applying a cold compress to soothe the skin can help reduce any lingering redness or mild swelling. It's best to steer clear of makeup or any heavy skincare products for at least 24 hours to allow the skin to recover naturally.

Gentle cleansing and moisturizing are key in the days following RF treatment. Use a mild, fragrance-free cleanser and apply a lightweight moisturizer to keep your skin hydrated. Avoid exfoliating products, retinol, or any strong acids for at least a week, as they can cause further irritation. Patting (not rubbing) the skin dry after cleansing is also essential to avoid further sensitivity.

In addition to at-home care, spacing out RF sessions properly is crucial for optimal results. While RF sessions don't typically have downtime, it's recommended to wait at least 2-4 weeks between treatments. This allows the collagen in your skin to rebuild, which contributes to tighter, firmer skin. Consulting with your specialist on timing for follow-ups can help maintain improvements without risking over-stimulation of your skin.

Best Skincare Products For Post-RF Care

Choosing the right skincare products for post-RF care can make a big difference in your skin's recovery and appearance. Look for products that focus on hydration and repair, such as hyaluronic acid serums, which help attract moisture to the skin, keeping it plump and reducing dryness. Peptide-rich creams are also excellent for enhancing collagen production, which is vital after RF treatments, as they help support the skin's healing process.

In addition to hydrating products, calming ingredients like aloe vera, chamomile, and allantoin can help soothe the skin and reduce any redness or irritation. Vitamin C serums, while helpful for brightening skin and supporting collagen, should be used with caution. It's best to wait a few days after RF before incorporating Vitamin C back into your routine to avoid potential sensitivity.

Avoiding harsh ingredients like retinoids and acids for about a week post-treatment is recommended to prevent irritation. Incorporating a gentle, fragrance-free moisturizer twice daily will also protect your skin's natural barrier and keep it balanced. Always follow with sunscreen to prevent any sun-related skin issues, as your skin will be more sensitive to UV exposure after RF treatments.

The Role Of Moisturizers And Sunscreen

Moisturizers and sunscreen are essential components of post-RF care, as they provide the hydration and protection your skin needs to heal and maintain results. Applying a gentle, hydrating moisturizer twice a day helps lock in moisture, which can be particularly beneficial after RF treatment, as the skin may feel drier? Look for ingredients like ceramides, hyaluronic acid, and squalane, which support the skin's barrier and reduce sensitivity.

Sunscreen is equally important, as RF treatments can make your skin more sensitive to the sun. Choose a broad-spectrum sunscreen with an SPF of at least 30 and ensure it's non-comedogenic and fragrance-free. Reapply every two hours if you're outdoors to protect the skin from harmful UV rays that can cause damage and reverse the benefits of RF treatment.

To maximize effectiveness, apply moisturizer first and then sunscreen as the last step of your skincare routine before going out. Avoid using chemical sunscreens immediately post-RF, as these may irritate; instead, opt for physical or mineral-based sunscreens with zinc oxide or titanium dioxide. This combination of moisturizer and sunscreen will help protect, nourish, and maintain your skin's new glow.

How Diet And Hydration Affect RF Results

Maintaining a balanced diet and staying hydrated play essential roles in supporting RF treatment results. Drinking sufficient water, typically eight glasses a day helps flush out toxins and keeps the skin plump and hydrated. When skin is well-hydrated, collagen production is more efficient, which can enhance the tightening and smoothing effects of RF.

Including protein-rich foods in your diet is also beneficial, as collagen is a protein. Foods like lean meats, fish, eggs, and legumes can support your body's natural collagen production, which is crucial for skin elasticity and firmness. Additionally, consuming antioxidants from fruits and vegetables can help protect your skin from environmental stressors and aid in the healing process.

Avoid excessive sugar and highly processed foods, as they can lead to glycation, a process that damages collagen. By maintaining a balanced diet rich in nutrients and antioxidants, you'll support both the immediate and long-term results of your RF skin tightening treatments, allowing you to enjoy firmer, more radiant skin over time.

Frequency Of Follow-Up Sessions For Lasting Effects

The frequency of follow-up RF skin tightening sessions varies based on factors like age, skin type, and individual goals. For most individuals, treatments every 2-4 weeks provide optimal results, as this frequency allows enough time for the skin to heal and new collagen to form. Initial treatment plans might include a series of 4-8 sessions, followed by maintenance treatments every few months to retain results.

After completing the initial sessions, discuss a personalized maintenance plan with your provider. Monthly or quarterly sessions can help sustain improvements, as RF effects tend to build gradually over time. Those looking for more substantial results or dealing with deeper wrinkles may benefit from more frequent touch-ups, though it's essential to avoid overdoing it to prevent skin fatigue.

Sticking to a consistent schedule helps reinforce collagen production, which in turn, contributes to a smoother, firmer complexion. Regular sessions, paired with a solid skincare regimen, can help you enjoy the benefits of RF treatments longer and maintain youthful, vibrant skin.

Avoiding Sun Exposure And Other Skin Stressors

Sun exposure and other environmental factors can significantly impact RF treatment results, as treated skin becomes more vulnerable to UV damage. Avoid direct sun exposure, especially in the first week after treatment, to prevent any potential side effects such as pigmentation issues. When going outside, wear protective clothing like wide-brimmed hats and long sleeves to shield treated areas.

In addition to avoiding the sun, it's essential to stay away from hot environments like saunas, steam rooms, or hot tubs for at least a few days post-treatment.

Excessive heat can cause inflammation and irritation, delaying recovery and affecting results. Similarly, avoid rigorous exercise immediately after RF, as sweat and heat can contribute to skin sensitivity and discomfort.

Environmental pollutants and smoking can also impair skin health and reduce RF treatment effectiveness. Using a barrier repair moisturizer, such as one with antioxidants, can help shield your skin from pollutants. By reducing exposure to these stressors, you'll support healthier, more resilient skin and preserve the tightening effects of your RF treatment longer.

CHAPTER NINE

Common Concerns And FAQS

When considering radio frequency (RF) skin tightening, it's essential to address common concerns and questions. Many individuals worry about potential side effects or discomfort during the treatment.

Generally, RF treatments are well-tolerated, but some patients may experience mild redness or swelling post-procedure. It's important to discuss any specific concerns with a qualified practitioner, who can provide tailored advice based on your skin type and health history.

Another common concern revolves around the number of sessions required for optimal results. Typically, most individuals need a series of treatments spaced a few weeks apart to achieve their desired outcome. Your practitioner will assess your skin condition and recommend a personalized treatment plan, ensuring you have a clear understanding of the process and timeline involved.

Lastly, many people question whether RF skin tightening is a suitable option for them. While RF is generally safe for a wide range of skin types, specific medical conditions or medications may affect your candidacy. Consulting with a skincare professional is crucial, as they can evaluate your skin and provide tailored recommendations to help you make an informed decision.

How Long Does RF Skin Tightening Results Last?

The longevity of results from RF skin tightening can vary from person to person, typically lasting anywhere from six months to two years. Factors such as age, skin condition, and lifestyle habits significantly influence how long the effects endure. Following the recommended treatment regimen, including maintenance sessions, can help extend the results.

To maximize the duration of your results, maintaining a good skincare routine post-treatment is essential. This includes using high-quality moisturizers, sunscreen, and products rich in antioxidants. Additionally, staying hydrated and adopting a healthy lifestyle can contribute to the longevity of your tightened skin, ensuring you reap the benefits for as long as possible.

Regular follow-ups with your skincare provider can help monitor your skin's condition and suggest when maintenance treatments might be beneficial. Staying proactive about your skin health will not only preserve the results but also promote overall skin vitality and elasticity.

Can RF Be Used On All Skin Types?

RF skin tightening is generally considered safe for all skin types, including sensitive and darker skin tones. Unlike other procedures, such as laser treatments, RF technology does not rely on light, which can be less effective or potentially harmful to certain skin types. The RF energy targets the deeper layers of the skin, promoting collagen production without significant surface damage.

However, individuals with specific skin conditions, such as active acne or severe skin infections, may need to avoid RF treatments until their skin heals. Consulting with a qualified skincare professional will help determine if RF is the right option for you. They will conduct a thorough assessment, including skin type analysis and medical history review, to ensure the best outcomes.

Before the treatment, your provider will discuss your skin type and any concerns you may have. They can also offer personalized recommendations on how to prepare your skin for the procedure, ensuring you achieve optimal results while minimizing risks.

Is RF Safe For The Eye And Neck Areas?

RF skin tightening can be safely performed on various areas of the body, including the neck and around the eyes. The technology is designed to deliver controlled energy to the skin, stimulating collagen production and tightening the skin without causing damage. Practitioners often use specialized techniques and lower energy settings when treating sensitive areas, ensuring comfort and safety.

During treatment, your provider will take extra precautions to protect your eyes, often using goggles or eye shields. It's essential to choose a qualified and experienced practitioner who understands the nuances of treating delicate areas, as they will tailor the approach to your specific needs and skin type.

Post-treatment care is also crucial for sensitive areas like the neck and around the eyes. Following your provider's aftercare instructions can help minimize any potential side effects and ensure you achieve the best possible results from your RF skin tightening session.

Will RF Skin Tightening Work For Sagging Skin?

RF skin tightening is particularly effective for addressing sagging skin by stimulating collagen and elastin production in the deeper layers of the dermis. The heat generated during the treatment encourages skin tightening and lifting, making it a popular choice for individuals experiencing mild to moderate skin laxity. While results may vary based on skin condition and individual factors, many clients see noticeable improvements in firmness and elasticity after a series of treatments.

For optimal results, it's often recommended to combine RF skin tightening with a holistic skincare approach. This may include maintaining a healthy diet, staying hydrated, and using products that support skin health, such as those rich in vitamins and antioxidants. Additionally, following your practitioner's advice regarding the number of sessions required will ensure the best outcomes.

It's important to have realistic expectations; while RF can significantly improve the appearance of sagging skin, it may not completely replace more invasive procedures like facelifts. However, many patients appreciate RF as a non-surgical option that offers visible results with minimal downtime.

Costs And Affordability Of RF Treatments

The cost of RF skin tightening treatments can vary widely based on several factors, including the provider's expertise, location, and the specific technology used. On average, a single session may range from $200 to $600, with packages for multiple sessions often available at a discounted rate. It's essential to discuss pricing with your provider upfront and understand what is included in the treatment plan.

Insurance typically does not cover RF skin tightening, as it is considered an elective cosmetic procedure. However, many clinics offer financing options or payment plans to help make treatments more accessible. Researching different providers and comparing costs can also help you find a solution that fits your budget.

While cost is an important consideration, focusing solely on price can be misleading. The experience and qualifications of the practitioner should also weigh heavily in your decision. Choosing a reputable provider ensures that you receive safe, effective treatments and satisfactory results.

CHAPTER TEN

Expert Tips For Best Results

To achieve the best results from radio frequency (RF) skin tightening, consistency is key. Regular treatments spaced according to professional recommendations allow the collagen in your skin to gradually build, providing firmer, smoother skin. Most people see noticeable improvements after 6 to 12 sessions, but the exact number varies based on individual skin types and goals. Be patient, as the skin's natural regeneration process can take time.

Hydration plays a vital role in RF skin tightening. Drinking plenty of water before and after your sessions ensures that your skin remains hydrated, which aids in the effectiveness of the treatment. Dry skin might not respond as well, so make sure to use moisturizers rich in hyaluronic acid or glycerin to keep your skin in optimal condition.

Finally, avoid excessive sun exposure before and after treatments. Sun damage can counteract the effects of RF, so use a high-SPF sunscreen daily to protect your skin. This not only prolongs your results but also prevents premature aging.

Combining RF With Other Skin Treatments

For enhanced results, radio-frequency skin tightening can be combined with other treatments like microneedling, chemical peels, or LED light therapy. Microneedling boosts collagen production, complementing RF by allowing deeper penetration of energy into the skin. This combination can yield faster and more dramatic results for those looking to tighten and rejuvenate their skin.

Chemical peels work well with RF as they exfoliate dead skin cells, allowing the radio frequency to work more efficiently on fresher skin layers. However, it's essential to space these treatments out adequately, allowing your skin time to heal between each session. Always consult with a professional to determine the best treatment schedule for your skin.

LED light therapy is another popular treatment to pair with RF. While RF focuses on tightening the skin, LED helps to calm inflammation, reduce redness, and promote healing. Together, these treatments can target different skin concerns simultaneously, offering a more comprehensive anti-aging routine.

Maintaining Skin Elasticity Between Treatments

Between radio frequency treatments, it's important to maintain the skin's elasticity with proper care. One of the best ways to do this is by applying skincare products containing peptides and retinol. Peptides help to boost collagen and elastin production, while retinol accelerates cell turnover, keeping the skin smooth and firm.

Exercise and a balanced diet also play a role in maintaining skin elasticity. Regular workouts increase circulation, delivering essential nutrients to your skin, while a diet rich in antioxidants, vitamins, and healthy fats keeps the skin nourished. Foods like salmon, avocados, and leafy greens are excellent for supporting skin health from within.

Lastly, be mindful of your lifestyle habits. Avoid smoking and excessive alcohol consumption, as both can degrade collagen and elastin fibers. Staying well-hydrated and getting enough sleep also helps to preserve the skin's natural firmness, making the effects of your RF treatments last longer.

Skincare Routine Adjustments For RF Users

If you're undergoing RF skin tightening treatments, it's important to make some adjustments to your skincare routine.

In the days leading up to and following your treatment, avoid using harsh exfoliants, retinoids, or acid-based products like glycolic or salicylic acid. These can irritate the skin and make it more sensitive to the RF energy.

After each session, focus on soothing and hydrating your skin. Use products with calming ingredients like aloe vera, chamomile, or Centella Asiatica. Hyaluronic acid serums are particularly beneficial for keeping your skin plump and hydrated post-treatment. Sunscreen is non-negotiable; apply a broad-spectrum SPF 30 or higher daily, even when indoors.

For the long term, incorporate anti-aging products that work in tandem with RF treatments. Vitamin C serums help protect the skin from free radicals and improve the effectiveness of the RF process, while products containing peptides or collagen can further boost skin tightening results.

Best Practices For Long-Lasting Youthful Results

To maintain long-lasting results from RF skin tightening, regular maintenance sessions are crucial. Even after you've completed your initial treatment plan, most dermatologists recommend follow-up sessions every 4 to 6 months to sustain the results. This keeps collagen production active, preventing sagging and fine lines from returning.

In addition to in-office treatments, at-home RF devices can be used to complement professional treatments.

While they aren't as powerful, they provide a gentle maintenance option between sessions. When used consistently, they help to prolong the results of clinical RF treatments.

Daily skincare habits also play an important role. Always cleanse and moisturize your skin, and apply sunscreen diligently. Avoid behaviors that damage collagen, such as tanning beds or smoking, and incorporate antioxidant-rich products into your routine to fight free radicals that age your skin over time.

Top Tips From Dermatologists And RF Technicians

Dermatologists and RF technicians stress the importance of customizing your treatment plan based on your skin type and concerns. For those with sensitive skin, they often recommend a slower approach with fewer, more spaced-out sessions to minimize irritation. For thicker skin, more frequent treatments may be necessary to achieve noticeable results.

They also advise against overdoing RF treatments. More isn't always better; too many treatments can lead to skin irritation or adverse effects. Stick to a plan guided by a professional, and don't rush the process. Your skin needs time to regenerate between sessions.

Lastly, always choose a licensed and experienced provider for RF skin tightening. Poorly administered treatments can result in burns or uneven results. A qualified technician will not only ensure your safety but will also provide personalized advice on how to get the most out of your RF treatments.

Conclusion

In conclusion, radio frequency (RF) skin tightening is a popular, non-invasive cosmetic procedure that offers a promising solution for individuals seeking to improve skin elasticity and combat signs of aging.

By utilizing RF energy, this technique stimulates collagen and elastin production in the deeper layers of the skin, leading to firmer, smoother, and more youthful-looking skin over time. This treatment has become a preferred alternative to surgical options because of its minimal downtime, reduced risk, and natural-looking results.

RF skin tightening is versatile and effective for a wide range of skin types and areas, including the face, neck, arms, abdomen, and thighs. The non-invasive nature of RF allows individuals to resume daily activities almost immediately post-treatment, making it convenient for those with busy lifestyles. Results generally appear over several weeks or months as collagen production continues, with peak effects often visible after multiple sessions.

The safety and efficacy of RF skin tightening have been widely documented, but success largely depends on factors such as skin type, age, lifestyle, and adherence to post-treatment care. While side effects are usually minimal and temporary, including mild redness or swelling, it's crucial to choose an experienced provider who can tailor the treatment to individual needs.

Ultimately, radio-frequency skin tightening represents a significant advancement in anti-aging aesthetics, offering an effective and less invasive route to rejuvenated skin. As technology continues to improve, RF treatments are becoming more targeted and efficient, allowing more people to achieve their desired results without surgical intervention. For anyone seeking to improve skin tone, texture, and firmness, RF skin tightening is a compelling option worth exploring, with results that can be both rewarding and confidence-boosting.

THE END

9 798300 533076